Veggies Not Included

Tales of a Triple Digit Weight Loss
from the Fast Food Lane

Christine Leo

Copyright © 2014 Christine Leo

All Rights Reserved. This book may not be reproduced, transmitted, or stored in whole or in part by any means, including graphic, electronic, or mechanical without the express written permission of the author, except by reviewers who may quote brief excerpts in connection with a review.

Published by: Christine Leo

Christine@ChristineLeo.com
www.ChristineLeo.com
www.VeggiesNotIncluded.com

Author: Christine Leo
Editor: Sandra Wendel, Write On, Inc.

This book is not intended as a substitute for the medical advice of a physician. You should not undertake any changes in your diet or exercise recommended in this book before consulting your personal physician. Neither the author nor the publisher shall be responsible or liable for any loss or damage allegedly arising as a consequence of your use or application of any information or suggestions contained in this book. You should regularly consult a physician in matters relating to your health and particularly with respect to any symptoms that may require diagnosis or medical attention.

Edition: May 2014

ISBN-13: 978-1500186302
ISBN-10: 1500186309

To my mom, who passed away while this book was being edited.

Look Mom, I did it! The book is finally finished. I'm so glad I got to read parts of it to you. Thank you for always being my biggest supporter. It was through your example of fierce determination that I never gave up. Thank you for always believing in me, often more than I believed in myself. I miss you more than I thought was humanly possible.

Love,
Your Chris

P.S. I went back to the title you liked.

TABLE OF CONTENTS

Introduction

1. The Naked Truth about My Wake-Up Call	1
2. The Big Secret: Most Diets Work	5
3. The Wonder (Bread) Years	10
4. My Descent to Rock Bottom	15
5. Get Your Head in the Game	20
6. Foodology: Would You Like Fries with That Weight Loss?	25
7. The Physical Transformation from Hungry to Satisfied	35
8. Just the Food Facts	40
9. The Emotional Transformation: Confessions of a Food Addict	54
10. The Whole Big (But Getting Smaller) Picture	58
11. The Lighter Side	63
12. Yes, There's Life after Losing	68

About the Author

INTRODUCTION

Dear Reader,

I lost 130 pounds.

Is that the most important part?

Nope.

What really matters is *why*. Why did I decide to change my life? Why was this time different? And why have I been able to keep the weight off for years now?

The "why" is especially important when you consider that I wasn't just heavy for a fraction of my life. I've been overweight my *entire* life.

At the risk of sounding sacrilegious, my goal with this book is not really to inspire you, but rather to take the entire subject of weight loss out of the clouds. I want to demystify, debunk and deflate the elusive enigma of losing weight that so many have put on a pedestal.

The "so many" I'm referring to are the media, weight loss companies, health experts and even fellow dieters. My greatest wish is that this book will get you into a headspace where you can actually believe that losing weight—and keeping it off—*is possible!*

After reading quite a few weight loss memoirs, I have found that most fall into one of two categories: "The Coach" and "The Blogger." Coaching memoirs read like how-to manuals, with a side of "Go get 'em, tiger!" and no real insight into the author's internal struggles. Other memoirs are like a never-ending blog, where the author falls short of giving the reader basic details about the tools the blogger used to attain success. I hope this book strikes a balance between the two.

Before I go any further, I would like to point out that this is a memoir. I am *not* a medical professional. I have a desk job just like many of you. I am here to share my story and the gritty details of how I did it. Please use common sense and consult your physician before taking on any weight loss plan.

I hope you find some workable strategies, enjoy my story, and get a few laughs along the way.

The Naked Truth about My Wake-Up Call

I fell off the gynecologist's exam table, buck naked.

No, this wasn't rock bottom. It turns out rock bottom wasn't some blaringly obvious single moment in time. You weren't going to find me passed out in sloppy pajamas lying face down in a sea of candy wrappers. For me, rock bottom was a series of uncomfortable, emotionally painful moments that drove me head first into a state of mind so raw, so focused, that it would become my secret weapon against overeating.

It was January 2008, approximately one month before my wedding, and I was on a quest for birth control. I was 25 years old and had an appointment with a new gyno. I had only been through one other female exam in my life, and aside from the humiliation of being spread eagle for someone I had just met, it hadn't been a complete train wreck.

When I entered the medical office and approached the front counter, I noticed the little window the receptionist sat behind was closed. After standing there awkwardly for a few seconds, another female patient looked up from flipping through a magazine and said, "You're going to have to knock on the window, honey."

"Oh. Thanks," I said, thinking that was strange. *Were they going to ask me for a secret password, like "cervix," too?*

I barely tapped on the window when it snapped open, revealing a dark-haired woman.

"Yes?" The woman asked in a clipped tone, keeping the "What the hell do you want?" part to herself.

"Hi, this is my first time here. I have an appointment."

"Did you sign in?"

I looked around to see if there was a clipboard on my side of the window.

"There's no …"

"Here," she said and pushed the clipboard at me from her side of the porthole.

I wasn't sure if the receptionist was frustrated with herself for not realizing that *she* was the actual possessor of the clipboard or with me for occupying her airspace.

I begin filling out my name when she barked, "Insurance?" I stopped what I was doing to fumble through my purse to find my wallet.

A second later, the receptionist let out a heavy sigh and said, "Let me know when you get it together," and slammed the window shut.

Now, some people might refer to this as an "Oh, hell no!" moment.

I, on the other hand, didn't possess an ounce of self-respect at the time. Combine that with an affinity for avoiding confrontation like the bubonic plague and, voila, you have yourself a genuine doormat.

I was a painfully sweet, overly nice, never confrontational, always apologetic, self-effacing people pleaser. You could practically break my arm, and I would still never own up to having a personal preference. I would go *any*where, do *any*thing for *any*one at *any* time.

The problem with that? It was all a big, fat lie! The energy it took to keep up the façade was slowly wearing me down. The only thing quieting my internal struggle was—of course, you guessed it—FOOD!

I entered the doctor's exam room thinking the worst was over. I got naked, hopped up on the table and used the two paper towels they gave me to cover my ladyparts the best I could. As I sat there, I noticed the stirrup-end of the table was facing a giant frosted glass window.

Really? Was this a sick joke? Did the gyno want to make sure we felt extra naked or something?

If so, mission accomplished. I could actually see the silhouette of a man talking on his cell phone outside in the courtyard.

I was fighting the urge to put my clothes back on when Dr. Sensitivity, herself, entered the room. She mumbled some kind of an introduction and then proceeded to bark questions at me in a staccato similar to the pit bull who was running the front desk.

"Why didn't you put down the date of your last cycle?" Dr. S. asked.

"It was a couple of weeks ago and I don't know the exact date."

Dr. S. ripped a calendar off the wall and thrust it into my hands. "Pick a date. We won't move forward until you do."

At this point, I started trying to plan an exit strategy. Unfortunately, I was naked and realized anything I could concoct would involve a high level of awkwardness. So I opted to stay the course in the name of contraceptives.

By the time I was on my back, Dr. S. was slapping my upper thigh and insisting I wasn't close enough to the end of the table.

"Closer! Come closer," she shouted.

I was already at the end of the exam table, but being the placating gal that I was, I scooted farther down until my butt was hanging over the edge.

When Dr. S. turned around briefly, I used the opportunity to push against the stirrups to try to wiggle myself back up onto the table just a smidgen. That's when one of my sock-covered feet lost traction, slipped from the stirrup and the momentum pulled me from the table.

Yes, I hit the floor, buck naked, punctuated by the fleshy sound of my butt smacking the cold hard tile.

I scrambled from the floor and back into the saddle as quickly as I could.

Dr. S. actually looked irritated with me. As if I had done it on purpose. After a few awkward apologies on my part, Dr. S. got on with the exam and everything seemed to be fine until I asked her about birth control.

She laughed. "I can prescribe them, but they probably won't work. You're too heavy! You need to lose weight first," she said.

"But I'm getting married in less than a month."

"Then I would suggest learning to enjoy yourself using condoms."

I felt as if someone had thrown a bucket of ice water on me.

A Teachable Moment

I may have left the office that day without a single shred of dignity intact, but I discovered something much more valuable—the tender beginnings of a backbone. For the first time in my life, I didn't walk away from the sting of humiliation, crying my eyes out while feeling sorry for myself. *I was pissed!*

Yes, I was mad at the doctor and her staff for the way they had treated me, but even more so at myself for allowing it to happen. I had spent my whole life so fearful people wouldn't like me that I'd take whatever crap was thrown my way lying down, like a good little victim.

However, this time was different.

The entire experience was a hard dose of reality, a wake-up call demonstrating just how little I valued myself. The girl who had spent years being pushed around finally understood the simple, yet foreign concept that if I didn't learn to respect myself first, no one else would.

The Big Secret: Most Diets Work

Before you call me insane and stop reading, think about it for a moment: most diets work. Think about all the late-night infomercials and advertisements for a weight loss product or program you've seen. Now try to think of one that *didn't* contain a success story or "before-and-after" photos.

Why is it that some diets work for others and not us? Why can Mary in Iowa lose 100 pounds on one of those celebrity-fronted weight loss programs, while you've joined the same program six times and can't lose more than 20 pounds? Why can Larry from accounting go on a low-carbohydrate diet and lose 50 pounds, yet you can barely part with the croutons on your chicken Caesar salad?

The answer is simple—Mary and Larry just found what worked for them.

Whenever I hear people say, "I've tried everything, but nothing works," what I actually hear is, "I've tried some stuff, but nothing I'm willing to commit to for the long haul."

On July 3, 2008, I decided I wanted to change my life *for good*. I was tired of watching people try to lose weight through Herculean efforts and give up or worse yet—succeed, just to gain it all back. When I stopped to really think about *why* people didn't stick with their chosen diet programs, it suddenly made perfect sense.

Often, when people choose to go on a weight loss program, their decision is made in haste. They are either chasing the promise of rapid weight loss through some fad diet or they are inspired by someone else's recipe for success and they're hoping to re-create it.

The problem with making a decision based on what others are doing is that it leaves out one key factor—YOU!

I knew that in order to lose weight and keep it off permanently, the road to success needed to be something I could live with for the long haul. Therefore, I made a revolutionary decision. I was going to factor my actual preferences into the equation. I knew that no matter what path I chose, I would be making sacrifices, but which sacrifices was I willing to make?

I'm going to be a diet rebel here and tell you that I lost nearly half my body weight while avoiding exercise and vegetables. Why? Because I really don't like either one of them. I would rather forgo a meal than spend an hour on a treadmill each day. I'd also rather eat an ice cream cone than five helpings of vegetables, even though I know vegetables are complex carbohydrates that will keep me fuller, longer.

That's why I chose calorie counting. At the end of the day, losing weight is all about calorie deficiency (in other words, burning more calories than I consume). Hence, I lost weight by eating 1,200 to 1,500 calories a day of foods I actually *wanted* to eat—like cheeseburgers and ice cream.

Don't believe me? I've got bank statements showing that I go to fast food chains every day. I can give you the names and numbers of at least ten people I eat with on a regular basis who will tell you I eat junk food.

I'm not telling you this to discourage you from eating healthy foods and exercising. On the contrary, if those are things you can work into your new lifestyle and stick with, wonderful! However, the thought of committing to vegetables, lean meats and exercise made me want to give up before trying. Call it a nicotine patch for the overweight, but turning my back on my own preferences felt like an equation for failure.

My goal was to create a path to success, and if that path didn't contain foods that were familiar, I wasn't going to stick with it. No amount of hypothetical willpower was going to change that. I've seen far too many people in my personal life lose 50-plus pounds the "right way" just to gain it all back in less than a year.

To those who would say that what I am proposing violates all tenets of good nutritious behavior, I say, perhaps. But according to whom? The same medical doctors who were writing prescriptions for weight loss pills, such as Fen-Phen back in the 1990s? That once-popular combo obesity drug is now banned because it caused heart valve problems. Or how about the doctors today who recommend bariatric surgeries for people who are only 80 to 100 pounds overweight?

Why will the same doctors who preach to you about the food guide pyramid also recommend you take these costly, sometimes harmful measures?

Because the medical community for years has been sending us the same bottom-line message: *Get the weight off!*

Light Bulb Time

How many of us know "naturally thin" people who seem to eat fast food all the time but never gain a pound? I used think they were either just lucky or lying through their teeth about how much exercise they actually did, but then a trip to a local hamburger joint with my two thin sisters-in-law opened my eyes.

We each ordered our food, and when we sat down at a booth, I had a double cheeseburger, fries and a chocolate shake on my tray. In contrast, they each had a single hamburger (no cheese), water and planned to share their order of fries. My lunch was 1,700 calories, while each of theirs was approximately 500 calories. There was no big secret. They hadn't made some magical deal with the fast food gods. They were eating the same style of food I was, but less of it.

That same night I went home and watched a report on the local news regarding the growing number of people having bariatric surgeries. They followed the story of a woman who, ironically, was around the same age, height and weight as me (mid-twenties, 5 feet 7 inches tall and almost 300 pounds). She underwent surgery and lost 100 pounds in less than six months.

The surgery cost her thousands of dollars, and she could only eat between 600 and 1,000 calories a day. It saddened me to think that someone my size was enduring a costly surgery just to force herself to eat fewer calories.

Not helping the situation is the fact that the celebrities who have undergone these surgeries are too busy smiling for the camera and talking about how they love their new bodies to explain some of the potential down sides. Weight loss surgeries can lead to gallstones, fecal/urinary incontinence and my personal favorite, "dumping syndrome."

Dumping syndrome occurs when undigested food bypasses the stomach and enters into the small intestine. This usually happens in gastric bypass patients who chew their food insufficiently or eat too much food at once. This leads to a host of food poisoning–like symptoms, including shaking, sweating, dizziness, extreme nausea, cramping, vomiting and diarrhea.

It's truly upsetting when people accuse my surgical weight loss brothers and sisters of taking the "easy way out." Trust me, they took the harder road. My new lifestyle is based on self-induced sacrifices that still afford me the occasional lapse in dietary judgment. They chose a path of forced sacrifices. For better or for worse, they have changed the internal structure of their physical body. They have no choice but to abide by their new body's limitations or face consequences.

After all this, I saw the light. Screw surgeries and the bombastic dieting ideals that lead to short-term successes or vomiting parties. I decided I was going to eat the same food I always had, but just less of it. If worse comes to worst, I stay the same size, but if best comes to better, I would get to lose weight and eat the foods that I enjoy.

The Wonder (Bread) Years

Cynicism can come in all shapes and sizes. Apparently, a chubby eight-year-old girl is one of them.

"Mom, I'm fatter than all the other girls on the drill team," I said.

My mom stopped scrubbing dishes long enough to look at me. "No you're not, honey. Don't be ridiculous."

"*Yes, I am!* I'm the only one who needed an extra-large uniform."

Somehow, my mother, a single parent, had found the money for me to participate in my elementary school dance troop made up of third- and fourth-grade girls. We all got to wear makeup, shiny nylons and bells on our shoes. For prepubescent girls, this was the big time!

However, while all other little girls had fun, I was like a miniature body-typing Sherlock Holmes, looking for evidence that would support my "I'm bigger than everyone else" hypothesis.

My mother never responded to my comment that day. It looked as if she was about to say something, and then she stopped herself. Instead, she took a deep breath, said my nickname, "Chris," on a sigh and went back to scrubbing the dishes.

The fact of the matter is my mother had spent her whole life playing the physical and emotional "weight game" herself. To see her eight-year-old daughter struggling with it was devastating. She didn't know what to say to me because she hadn't solved the puzzle for herself yet either. She told me I was beautiful and smart on a regular basis, but somehow, that just wasn't enough.

I look back at these memories and am staggered that at eight years old I had the presence of mind to even be aware of such things. Secretly, it was one of the reasons I was terrified to have my own children. Why bring a new person into the world who will just start hating herself in a few short years? Why would I wish that existence on anyone, let alone, my own child?

What I didn't understand at the time is that this heightened sense of self-awareness was a learned behavior from the adults around me. And no, I'm not going to blame this solely on my mother. It takes a village, remember? I can recall countless extended family members, teachers, people at church, friends of the family and television shows all feeding me examples of self-recrimination.

Young children are not just sponges absorbing what you tell them, they're more like tofu, which will take on the flavor of whatever it is simmered in. It's not enough to simply *tell* your kids they're wonderful. You have to lead by example. You have to believe that you, yourself, are worthy of respect and love.

Lord of the Flies (aka Junior High)

Ah, yes, junior high. The time when puberty, bad hair and cliques converge making the popular, more popular while the rest of us become the steps upon which they rise to their meteoric high school greatness. If you don't know what I'm talking about, then you were either popular or traveled with a large enough posse that you were never trampled. To my fellow flattened classmates, I don't have to explain why this was the darkest time in my childhood.

In the two years it took to get through middle school, I had no less than five bullies who made harassing me their favorite pastime. They haunted me during classes, in between classes, during lunchtime and, of course, during physical education. I wasn't allowed to forget for even a millisecond that I was a fat ass, Free Willy, thunder thighs or big Bertha. One kid followed me around for a solid semester mooing and oinking at me whenever he saw me. Eventually, things got so bad that I started missing at least one day of school a week. I was constantly forging notes in my mother's handwriting just to get myself out of PE.

It was during these years that my food addiction hopped into the fast lane. I began to hide food and gorge when I was alone, which was easy to do because I was a latchkey kid. I would find whatever sugary morsel we had in the house and make it work to my advantage. If we had jelly and no bread, I'd smear it on a tortilla. If we had maple syrup, I quickly became a pancake connoisseur. When my mom was home, I would steal change out of her purse so I could race to the corner convenient store for anything with the name Little Debbie written across it.

What made junior high so much worse than any other time was the feeling of helplessness. I was finally becoming aware of the world in an adult-like way, but I was too young to escape the events that caused me pain. Honestly, if I attended a college or had a job where people harassed me the way bullies did in junior high, I would have left (and possibly been legally justified in pressing charges).

Welcome to Reality

During high school, real life kicked me in the ass. Actually, it kicked my whole family in the ass. The summer before I was supposed to begin my freshman year of high school, my mom lost her job and we were forced to move out of the small apartment we called home.

My mother, younger brother and I moved in with my aunt until we could get back on our feet. In the meantime, my mom enrolled me in a home-schooling program since we didn't know where we were going to end up. Six months later, we were sleeping on the floor of yet another tiny one-bedroom apartment with only a couple of mattresses and a refrigerator to our names.

Suddenly, my world expanded. The red curtain life's *real* problems hid behind dropped and, once again, I turned to food to help me cope. The same four years most teens are worried about clothes, friends, prom, driving and getting into a good college, I was playing homemaker and nanny to my little brother while my mother worked two jobs. High school became something I did through the mail, in between cooking dinner and ripping eviction notices off our door.

The emotional turmoil these years put me through turned me inside out. The anger, guilt, desperation, bitterness, sadness, loneliness and confusion I felt was like sludge that barely allowed me to move. I wish I could say I had some "inner strength" that got me through these rough times, but the truth is I had food to numb the pain. I gained over 100 pounds in high school, and when I emerged to enter college, I weighed nearly 260 pounds.

A Time of Learning

College was the first time I discovered what I could truly accomplish with a little self-belief. I discovered the direct connection between hard work, dedication and achieving things I had previously thought unattainable. It was also the first (and only other time) that I lost nearly 100 pounds.

I went on a low-carb diet at the age of 19 and dropped 90 pounds over the course of six months (I went from 260 pounds down to 167). The only problem: I wasn't *really* ready to lose the weight, not mentally or emotionally. I went on the diet after reading a book about the low-carb lifestyle and became excited about the prospect of losing weight while still getting to overeat one food group (protein). My success was extremely short lived. It took about two years, but the second I stopped eating low-carb, the weight came right back on, and then some.

This isn't me saying that low-carb dieting is bad. I just hadn't done the self-examination required to truly commit. I hadn't really hit rock bottom.

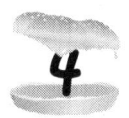

My Descent to Rock Bottom

MEAN PEOPLE SUCK!

No truer statement hath ever been composed.

Yet, if we are talking about mean people, I have to include myself in that line-up. Self-hatred is an insidious cancer, and while I could go on for days about all the people who made fun of me growing up, nobody was as cruel to me as I was to myself.

The truth is people with low self-esteem are some of the most self-centric people you will ever meet. Now, before you accuse me of blasphemy, allow me to explain. I didn't say we are an unkind, uncompassionate or unsupportive bunch. I just said we spend a lot of time and energy thinking about ourselves—in a negative way.

If I could quantify all the hours I spent inside my own head obsessed with how much I hated my body, I could have earned a doctorate. There were countless outings, birthdays, dates, graduations, weddings, and vacations—times for fun and celebration—where I can barely remember what happened because I was too busy hating how I looked to pay attention.

Much like when you have a pimple on your face and you're convinced that it's all anyone can see, I thought my weight was all anyone noticed about me. Even when I was just passing by a stranger in the grocery store, I was positive they were thinking, *Look, there goes a fat chick,* rather than trying to figure out what to feed their family for dinner that night.

This microscopic self-awareness led to a bunch of odd, spy-like behavior: Casing a room to see if I was the biggest one there, *never* making eye contact, avoidance of all photographic and video recording equipment, dressing in layers of black clothing even in the dead of summer, covertly hiding behind large purses, coats and hairdos. You get the point.

Almost to Rock Bottom

I said at the beginning of this book that for me, rock bottom was a series of uncomfortable, emotionally painful moments. Admittedly, the events that followed the gyno trip from hell weren't as bad, but they fueled my journey to rock bottom.

What three words will make any self-loathing big girl want to run for the hills?

Wedding. Dress. Shopping.

Most women would agree that if ever there were a time for "vanity sizing" (the practice of labeling larger clothing a size smaller) *this would be it!* Instead, most wedding dresses run two sizes too small. Oh joy! My one attempt at going to a real bridal boutique went something like this:

I walk into the store with my entourage feeling like a size zip code.

The Orange County Barbie doll working there approaches one of my skinnier friends and says, "What kind of wedding dress did you have in mind?"

My friends quickly correct her before I can say, "Yo, skinny bitch, over here."

The Barbie doll pastes a plastic smile on her plastic face and apologizes.

After playing along for a few minutes, I left the store without even trying on a dress.

What was the point? I already didn't want to traipse around in a wedding dress just to see my butt in a mirror from every angle known to man. Tip for people who work in bridal boutiques: When approaching a group full of women who just entered your store, try something like, "So who's the lucky girl?" Don't just walk up to the woman you *think* looks most like a bride and address her as such.

I ended up buying my wedding dress on eBay.

Pit Stop at Newlywed Central

The wedding day had come and gone, as well as the honeymoon. I should be happy, but there I sat, just a few months after marrying the love of my life, Googling the phrase "post-marital depression." Yet, none of the search results seemed to apply to me. Some articles talked about how it's a letdown to no longer be the center of attention. *Um, yeah, I don't think so!* Obviously, those articles weren't written for the 300 pound bride who would rather have a root canal, than go through a two-hour photo session.

Some articles hinted at the reality of marriage not meeting the expectation. There might have been some truth to this, but I had been with my husband for two years at this point. We knew each other's goods and bads. He was my best friend and there was no one else I would rather spend my life with… So, why wasn't I happy?

For the first time in my life, I had to admit that the problem was *not* external. It was easy to blame my depression and addiction to food on outside life when everything was in "turmoil," but for the first time, I was in a good place. I had finished my degree, found a great job and married the sweetest man I had ever met.

The true issue was that little thing called self-hatred, and its effects on my life were quickly growing larger than my waistline.

And We've Arrived

The bottom of the boulder was about six months after my wedding. It was my first business trip with a new job. I spent most of my time in an office, safe, behind three cubicle walls with a phone to my ear. I was never in front of people, shaking hands, standing on stages, and giving presentations.

This trip took me to one of the hottest places on earth. Okay, maybe I'm exaggerating, but it seriously reached 109 degrees while we were there. It involved a lot of running around outside, from one building to another, in professional attire (also known as, chafing polyester), while carrying boxes of supplies. I arrived at most of the events that week soaked in sweat and out of breath.

After perspiring my way through nearly every undergarment I had brought with me, I was sure it couldn't get worse.

Then I looked in the mirror.

I was getting ready for an evening event when I noticed my nose and cheeks were badly sunburned, and my eyes were completely bloodshot. I had somehow managed to contract a case of pink eye while I was there.

I wanted to put a bag over my head and disappear. So you can guess how thrilled I was when I got to the event that evening, thinking I was only going to help "set up," and I was told I would be on stage in front of 600 people handing out commemorative plaques. Oh, and just in case those 600 people couldn't see me clearly, not to worry, there was a Jumbotron screen overhead that would capture every detail.

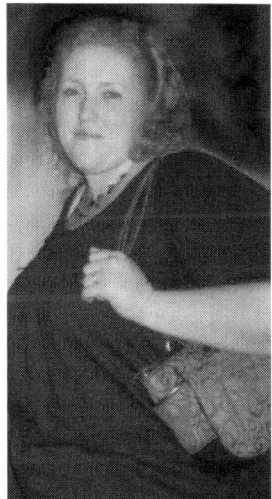

**The photo above was taken
that night in June 2008.**

Truthfully, was anyone really paying attention to what I looked like that night?

No, probably not.

Was it all in my head?

Yes, probably so.

But that was all it took. When it comes to self-perception, emotions *are* your reality. The pain you experience makes it real even if the facts don't.

My pain, embarrassment and shame had reached a boiling point and pushed me over the emotional edge. I finally discovered what was at rock's bottom and it was healthy dose of *FED UP!*

Get Your Head in the Game

I adore Celine Dion. She is a great example of getting your head in the game. No really, just go with me on this.

When Celine performs, she owns the stage. She plants her stilettos shoulder-width apart, pounds on her chest with a mighty fist and wails for all she's worth. It doesn't matter how eccentric she looks while doing it because at the end of the day, she gets the job done. She delivers.

She exemplifies my weight loss motto of "Whatever it takes!"

The reason for this motto is twofold: One, it reinforces my earlier statement that most weight loss programs work (it's just a matter of finding what works for you), and, two, it excuses some of the ugly places your mind might have to go in order to get your head in the game and keep it there.

I say "ugly places," because most of us are decent people who don't admire traits such as arrogance, selfishness and competitiveness. Yet, in a way, those are the very traits I had to embrace in order to keep myself focused for the entire year and a half it took me to lose the weight and then to keep it off.

Arrogance: "Failure is NOT an option!"

You can call it arrogance or sweeten it up by calling it confidence, either way, the result has to be the same for it to work. Be prepared to "fake it 'til you make it." You can't just "believe" you can lose the weight, you have to *know* you can! I realize how cheese-tastic this sounds, but there is power in the language we use.

I literally had to change my internal dialog. No more wishful statements such as, "*If* only I could lose this weight, I'd be so much happier." It became, "*When* I lose this weight, my ass is going to look killer in those jeans!"

I also changed my external dialog. My natural inclination was always to soften everything I said and never make confident statements about myself or my accomplishments, lest I sound arrogant. Oh, the horror!

Well, I got over it.

I forced myself to start using strong, definitive words and statements in place of fluffy, weaker ones. My new way of eating was *always* working (even when I was experiencing a plateau), and it was only a matter of time until I met my goal. I never left any room for question or argument as to the success of my weight loss. I was going to meet my goal!

This was more than me just trying to build my self-confidence. I was trying to build a foundation that would support my success. There were days when I wanted to fall off the wagon, and I needed something mentally sturdy to keep myself upright. I was angry for allowing myself to walk through life feeling like an outsider because of my size, so I let that anger fuel my determination to succeed. I no longer was willing to resign myself to an existence I hated.

Selfishness: "I'm not spending my calories on you!"

For those of us who have trouble sending cold soup back at a restaurant, this particular proclamation may be a bit of a challenge. In fact, I'm not going to be a hypocrite and tell you that I'm able to live by this diet-law all the time. This is about putting yourself before others. This is about telling the food-pushers of the world to "Back the hell off!" If you weren't aware that food is a personal thing, just try to tell a food-pusher, "No thanks, I'm good."

Them's fightin' words, son!

What a food-pusher really thinks you said is, "I didn't understand you the first time. Please offer me food again." Or "I don't like that particular kind of food. Please suggest something else." Or "I don't really care about your birthday, which is why I'm not eating cake."

If you are counting calories, carbs, fat grams, sodium or points and the item this person is offering you would derail your efforts, don't be afraid to say, "No thanks, I'm good." If that doesn't work, then make note that this person is a food-pusher, which means they equate your consumption of their edibles with your acceptance, respect and/ or affection for them, so a firmer hand is required.

When someone at the office brings cupcakes to celebrate a coworker's birthday, and you are not going to eat one, be nice at first and try to level with them. Tell them you are "on a diet" or "trying to change your life." If they don't back off or have the nerve to utter a phrase, such as "One bite won't hurt," then you have my permission to (1) Lay the verbal smack down, or (2) Take the passive road and say you have a stomach ache. *Whatever it takes!*

Competitiveness: "I'm going to prove you wrong!"

As you lose weight, you will inevitably encounter negative people. In fact, some will be downright mean, often veiling their insults in humor meant to bring you down.

It's bad enough that most of us have an inner voice of self-doubt that never shuts up. The last thing we need is to deal with negative comments from the outside world.

Personally, I've experienced everything from people pretending to make themselves vomit as if to imply I became bulimic in order to lose weight to comments like, "Oh, you finally decided to leave the Oreos alone, I see."

I'm here to tell you that their negative comments are about *them*, not about you. This isn't a case of you being "too sensitive" or "not having a sense of humor." It is a case of them being insensitive and having a cruel sense of humor.

So how do you deal with rejection? I suppose I could give you some bullshit advice to just ignore it, but last time I checked, we are human beings, not robots. If we hear or see something negative, chances are we are going to internalize it. So why fight the feeling? Internalize it and let their negativity fuel your drive to succeed. Prove them wrong!

The Difference Between Then and Now

This time I didn't lose weight because I wanted to be thin; I lost weight because I wanted my life to change. Aside from the embarrassment, shame and self-loathing, I was tired of not being able to function with the same freedom as others. Tired of asking for seat-belt extensions on planes. Tired of not being able to cross my legs. Tired of having to flip up the armrests at the movie theaters. Tired of wearing holes into my jeans because my thighs rubbed together. Tired of feeling as though I was going to pass out from walking up just one flight of stairs. The list goes on.

Unlike my last attempt at weight loss, this time my goal was reasonable. I knew I could achieve it, and, more importantly, I knew once I did, I would cherish it. The first time I lost nearly 100 pounds, my goal was to be thin. Sadly, I was never thin *enough*. I looked in the mirror after losing 100 pounds with the same level of disgust I had before.

This time I didn't permit the self-bashing. Instead of concentrating on how unhappy I was, I concentrated on the power I had to change it. That sounds deceivingly simple, but it's not. Self-belief cannot come after the weight loss. It must come before.

Foodology: Would You Like Fries with That Weight Loss?

Food is my saving grace.

It's funny how the very thing that once made me feel so out of control, made me feel in control while I was losing the weight. Food stopped being the source of my misery and became one of my tools for change.

Having a large amount of weight to lose is like staring down at the wide expanse of the Grand Canyon and knowing you have to cross it—on foot. As a product of the instant gratification generation, the last thing I wanted to hear about was patience. Unfortunately, there is no way around it. If you have 100-plus pounds to lose, it doesn't matter what path you choose, it's still going to take time.

With that said, food made me feel as if I was in the driver's seat. I knew where I wanted to go and that I could get there however fast or slowly I wanted based on the choices I made.

Step 1: What's in your caloric bank account?

If you go on a crazy shopping spree without knowing your credit limit first, you might be hit with an overdraft fee. In the game of eating, overdraft fees mean packing on the extra pounds. Our bodies burn a certain number of calories each day just to handle the regular internal functioning of our organs (such as our heart, lungs, kidneys, liver, nervous system and intestine). Knowing your number is power! It lets you know your body's tipping point for weight gain.

If you lead a sedentary lifestyle and eat the exact amount of calories it takes for your body just to function, you will remain at your current weight. Like a teeter-totter, if you eat more than that number of calories, you will gain weight, and if you eat less than that number, you will lose weight.

This magical number is called your Basal Metabolic Rate (BMR), not to be confused with BMI (Body Mass Index). There are tons of BMR calculators online, which will ask for your height, weight, age, gender and physical activity level.

When I first started out, my BMR was approximately 2,150 calories per day (I was 26 years old, 5 feet 7 and 300 pounds). By the way, that's assuming I am lying in bed all day. If I were to burn additional calories through any kind physical activity (from shopping to exercise), that just adds to the number of calories I can consume before I reach my body's weight gain tipping point.

Given that I worked a full-time job and ran plenty of errands, it's safe to say I was burning about 2,500 calories per day without intentional exercise. As I started changing my eating habits, I was only consuming 1,500 calories per day (at maximum), which means I was burning 1,000 calories a day. You have to burn a total of 3,500 calories to lose one pound. I was burning about 7,000 calories per week, equaling two pounds per week. In other words, I choose a daily caloric max that would allow me to lose about two pounds per week.

Did my actual experience fit these specific parameters exactly? No. My first month on the program (July 2008), I lost 17 pounds. I'm sure most of that was water. The months to follow, I lost approximately 10 pounds per month.

Step 2: Food Negotiations (aka What do you really want to eat?)

For me, this was an easy answer: I love junk food and I'm not a big fan of vegetables. Of course, there's more to it than that. You might think you love all food, but there are different levels of love. I like to think everyone has their "must haves," "negotiables" and "forgettables." To avoid your next meal becoming Sophie's Choice, create a list of foods, like I did, that you regularly flock to with the calorie counts noted, so you can reference it easily. Divide the food into the three categories described.

Despite my professed love of junk food, you might be surprised to find that I can live without potatoes (that means French fries, chips, mashed potatoes, hash browns, tater tots and their starchy relatives). That's not to say I don't like a French fry now and then, but I would forgo a side of McDonald's fries any day for one of their soft serve ice cream cones. In fact, I make that very tradeoff all the time, because I go to McDonald's just about every day. (Note: A small order of fries at McDonald's is 230 calories, but their soft serve cones are only 170 calories.)

Welcome to negotiations 101. I know some people might find this style of eating daunting, but it honestly has become second nature for me. Plus, in a day and age where you can get a phone app for everything from interpreting your dog's barks to building a virtual farm, the tools you need to track and research calories are literally at your fingertips.

Within a few weeks of regularly checking nutrition labels and websites for calorie counts, I was able to estimate the caloric content of most food. This style of eating kept me accountable in a way nothing else ever had before. It's funny how I enjoy a cookie more now than when I used to eat 20 in one sitting.

Overeating had a numbing, drugged out effect on me that is hard to explain. Sometimes it felt as if I wasn't even really tasting the food. Portion controlling cleared the cobwebs and forced me to face reality.

By the way, this is a good time to mention that if you happen to love fruits, vegetables, lean meats and whole grains, wonderful! Healthy foods are not just higher in nutrition, they are usually lower in calories, which means you can eat a greater quantity. They also take longer for your body to break down, which means you will be fuller, longer. Anytime you can forgo "junk food" for something healthy, without feeling deprived, go for it. More power to you. (Yes, I mean that whole-grain-heartedly.)

Step 3: Set the safety lock on trigger foods and activities.

"Triggers" usually refer to an external element that can provoke a behavior (whether desired or undesired). If you were an alcoholic, some obvious triggers would be alcoholic beverages and environments such as bars and parties where alcohol is present. Avoidance of triggers can be paramount to changing the behavior.

Now try that with food. You can't avoid the fact that you have to eat to live. However, with a little self-evaluation, it's possible to identify and avoid trigger foods and activities that you know will lead to overeating.

Remember that list I asked you to create? Well, I'm willing to bet that some of the foods listed in your "must haves" column aren't just foods you love, but they are foods that, when eaten, send you into a feeding frenzy. I suggest blacklisting those foods. Repeat after me, "They are not worth it." Believe me, nothing sucks more than gaining two pounds in one day when it took you a week to lose them. I realize this might sound contradictory coming from a woman who lost 130 pounds eating fast food, but a cheeseburger doesn't set me off. There are plenty of foods I have to abstain from.

Most of my trigger foods revolve around sugar such as donuts, pastries, sweet breads, brownies, pumpkin pie and cake. For me, there is no such thing as eating just one donut or being cute about it and cutting it in half. I absolutely go berserk. I will eat a half-dozen donuts in one sitting, an entire pie or a whole tray of brownies. Therefore, I don't touch them unless I'm absolutely prepared to go "all the way" and sacrifice the calories.

I've figured out what I can get away with and what I can't. For some reason, I can eat a small serving of ice cream or one cookie and walk away feeling satisfied. If you have foods you suspect might be a trigger, then experiment. Try to eat what the nutrition label says is a regular serving size and then walk away. You will know if it is a trigger food in less than five minutes.

Finally, be aware of activities and environments that make you want to overeat. For instance, cooking, watching others cook (on TV or in person) or going to a buffet all make me want to overeat. If I make a giant skillet of taco meat, I will inevitably consume more calories than if I just stop by Taco Bell and order one burrito. I don't frequent drive-thrus just because I like fast food, I do it because there is built-in portion control. They hand me a single serving of whatever I've ordered and I drive away.

Step 4: Find welcomed distractions.

In a roundabout way, Stephenie Meyer (author of the Twilight series) is responsible for helping me lose 30 pounds. I lost more weight in the two months it took me to complete the Twilight series than at any other time during my journey. It eventually dawned on me that maybe there was something to this, so I started using books to distract myself whenever I craved food.

Think of activities that you enjoy and become so immersed in you would be fine to go without food. That isn't to say that you couldn't eat during some of these activities, but if you're engaged enough, you won't miss food. Try hanging out with friends, shopping, reading, writing, video games, swimming, painting, fill in the blank.

If you don't have a passionate interest, maybe it's time you learn something new: Learn to speak a new language, take lessons to play an instrument, teach yourself to knit with YouTube videos, take a class at the community college … You get the idea.

Step 5: Create a game plan for success.

Now that you know how many calories you can consume each day without gaining weight, it's time to figure out how many you are willing to give up in order to lose. Remember, *you* are in the driver's seat. This is *your* car. You can take as little or as much time as you want to reach your destination. This is where I recommend you be kind to yourself.

Think about your food preferences and your willingness to negotiate. Sure, you can dive in head first, commit to eating an unrealistic 800 calories a day and lose 100 pounds in three months, but that's an insanely low calorie count unless you're a petite woman under five feet tall. Depriving yourself of the foods you love or an amount of food that keeps you sane is a bad idea! (A quick note: I will not entertain conversations about starving yourself. I do not advocate trading one eating disorder for another. This is about awareness, accountability, and portion control.)

Also, besides food preferences, take note of what times of the day you tend to eat most. Personally, I don't like eating breakfast in the morning and I tend to want to eat more at night. So I save my calories for the end of the day. I know, I know, here I go again, being a naughty dieter and telling you to do the exact opposite of what nutrition experts tell you to do.

In a perfect world, you should be eating a "hearty" breakfast because it gets your metabolism going and you will have the rest of the day to burn those calories off. If you happen to like large breakfasts and small dinners, then go for it!

You need to create in an environment for success. Most diets are so heavily geared toward what you *should* do, they rarely take into account what you *already* do. Yes, if you want to lose weight, you have to make some sacrifices. Does that mean you have to make stuff so miserable for yourself that you run screaming for the hills after two weeks? No!

Give yourself some concessions. If you are anything like I was, you have a Grand Canyon's worth of weight to lose, and right now your top priority should be sticking to the program. Pick and choose your battles. Take it one step at a time. If you want to be a dieting superhero, fine, but start out slowly.

If you can, plan the edible parts of your day. If you like to prepack your meals, great! This should be no problem for you. However, if you're like me and can't stand cooking and Tupperware, then think about where you will be getting lunch and dinner that day and plan what you will be selecting in advance.

Step 6: What to do when your game plan derails. Hello, Plan B!

This is one of the reasons I love calorie counting so much. Derailing can actually be a good thing.

On low-carb diets, eating an "accidental donut" is like undoing a week's worth of work. If you are following a low-carb diet, after three to five days of eating less than 30 to 50 grams of carbohydrates a day (the equivalent of two slices of white bread), your body will enter ketosis.

Ketosis is a state where, in the absence of carbohydrates, your body will begin to burn its stored fat for fuel. Now, before you start swearing off carbohydrates, those two pieces of bread I just mentioned would be off limits. As it turns out beef, poultry, eggs, cheese and of course, vegetables have some carbohydrates in them. Therefore, you will be reaching your daily allotment of carbs just by eating protein and some very select vegetables. There is no room for error on this diet. You don't start burning fat until day three (or later), and if you mess up, you have to start all over again to get your body back into ketosis.

As I said earlier, counting calories is like having a bank account, but the funds inside don't have to represent just one day's allotment of calories. Say you are trying to keep yourself on 1,500 calories a day and you "mess up" by eating 2,000 calories. You could eat just 1,000 calories the next day and then it was as if you ate 1,500 calories on both days. Similarly, if you had a little too much fun over the weekend, eating 3,000 calories on Saturday and 3,000 calories on Sunday, you could even the score by only eating 1,000 calories a day for the next six days. That would bring your average caloric intake for those eight days to 1,500.

Here's the reason this sort of "banking" is a good thing:

1. It keeps you accountable at all times. You will need to count your calories every day, even on days you mess up in order to use this methodology.
2. It has a built-in "stop-loss" mechanism. One of the reasons people fall off their diets and never get back on the horse is that once they have messed up, they figure, "What's the point. I've already gone this far. I'll just go back on the diet next week." If you have one bad day (or two or three), but you know you can correct the behavior in the days to come, you are less likely to put off your return to the diet indefinitely.
3. Messing up actually decreases your chance of plateauing. They call it calorie shifting. The idea is that if you were to eat the same number of calories each day,

your body becomes accustomed to burning off that number of calories. You can jump-start a complacent metabolism by eating heavily on one day and then dropping your caloric intake the next. Your metabolism will continue burning at a higher rate from the heavy day you had before, so when you suddenly eat lighter the next day, your metabolism is still burning at the high rate (thus burning more calories than usual). When I have a bad day, I just call it my calorie shifting day.

Step 7: How to keep the derailments to a minimum: What to do when a craving kicks in.

1. Stop! At this moment you're focused solely on your desire to eat (whether it's something specific or just anything). Calm down. Remind yourself you will be eating soon. Remember your next meal is only ___ minutes/ hours away. I realize this sounds stupid, but it works for me. I call it internal consoling. When you're about to go into a food frenzy, you need to use a voice of reason to take things down a notch.
2. Don't allow yourself to eat a snack if you know you're truly not hungry. If you try to eat a snack in this moment, that snack *will* turn into something more. You can't satisfy this moment with something small and reasonable.
3. Remind yourself *why* you are doing this. Expand your focus away from the moment. Fight to remind yourself why you started this journey (such as you were tired of feeling ashamed or tired of being unable to walk up stairs). Think back to the progress you've made on your journey and remind yourself that you should be building upon that, not taking steps back. If it helps, create a list of these reasons and keep it nearby.
4. Try one of the welcomed distractions such as reading or a hobby I discussed earlier.
5. Negotiate with yourself. If there is something you are "dying" to eat and you just can't let it go, then eat it—

but *after* your next meal. Play the role of responsible parent and make yourself wait until after your next meal to eat it. If possible, put it off until the next day. You might be surprised to find your desire for that particular food is not quite as strong as you think it is.
6. Forgive yourself. You are only human and you are trying to reverse (possibly a lifetime's worth of) destructive behavior. Call it a calorie shifting day and move on. Don't allow yourself to declare this single moment/ meal/ day/ weekend "diet Armageddon" and give up. This is one battle, not the war.

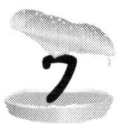

The Physical Transformation from Hungry to Satisfied

Aren't you hungry?
This was the number one question people would ask me after they found out exactly *how* I was losing weight. Initially, my answer was, "Yes." Why lie? I had spent far too much time speaking with people who acted as though they were God's gift to effective dieting, just to watch them gain it all back less than a year or two later.

If you can't tell by now, my perspective on weight loss is "Let's get real." The things you have to do to lose weight can suck. This is why I tried to make it suck less by getting real with myself early on in the game. The first couple of months of counting calories, I was hungry, but the important question was why was I hungry? It didn't take me long to realize that saving all my calories for one large meal a day was a stupid idea. Likewise, spending all my calories on something unsubstantial, such as the infamous donuts, would not sustain me throughout my day.

Counting calories did more than make me accountable for what went in my mouth. It made me hyperaware of my eating habits. Since I no longer allowed myself the luxury of gorging, I now had to eat with purpose.

I still ate small breakfasts and slightly larger dinners (as you will see from my meal examples in the next chapter), but when I did eat, it was with the intention of staving off hunger for as long as possible.

In the Beginning

I decided to start my new way of eating the day before the Fourth of July holiday in 2008. If you're wondering what the hell I was thinking starting a diet the day before a major holiday, I don't blame you. Looking back, I think my lack of concern over the holiday shows just how ready I was to make a change and that I wasn't about to let life events get in the way. I recall looking up the calories of typical foods you find at a barbeque in preparation for the holiday and planning accordingly.

During my first thirty days, I made the decision not to weigh myself. I knew my first weigh-in would be more impactful if I saw that I had lost a serious amount of weight. It's easy to quit a diet if you've only lost a few pounds. Twenty pounds is a different story.

In the first month, I lost 17 pounds. I remember jumping up and down shouting, "It's working! It's working!" It may have only been a drop in my weight loss bucket, but to have proof my efforts were paying off incentivized me to stay on track.

By the second month, I begin to share with my family and close friends what I was doing and how much progress I had made thus far. Almost everyone was supportive, but a few were not. I heard comments like, "Oh, anyone can lose 20 pounds" or "I can't count the number of times I've lost 20 pounds, and then gained it back." At the time, I couldn't process their negativity, so I decided I was either going to let their criticisms send me running back to the refrigerator or add it to my list of reasons to accomplish my goal.

I chose the latter.

Over the years, I've come to the realization that only the most insecure people would look at someone who has a long journey ahead of them and squash the little bit of hope that person was vulnerable enough to share with them. However, I'm eternally grateful that I was confronted by these patronizing attitudes because they fueled the fire in me to succeed like no amount of fat-shaming ever could.

It's a Miracle!

It took a while, but eventually my answer to "Aren't you hungry?" changed. I learned how to eat throughout my day so that my roaring appetite finally gave me a break and went on vacation. I got to where I could identify the difference between real hunger and artificial hunger (in other words, I could tell the difference between an empty stomach vs. hunger induced by a nice helping of stress).

Eventually, the wondrous miracle I had only heard about, but never before experienced, happened to me. I was about four months and 40 pounds into my weight loss, and my husband and I went to one of my favorite restaurants. I had decided ahead of time that this was going to be a calorie shifting day and I would let my hair down. I ordered a huge bacon cheeseburger and a side of steak fries. I got halfway through the burger and fries and … stopped. I literally could not eat another bite.

Ironically, that's when the gravity of the changes my body had been experiencing truly hit me. You would think the 40-pound weight loss would have done the trick, but, no, it was the fact that I couldn't finish a meal that just a few months ago I would have polished off with dessert.

The hardest part of my weight loss journey was not the occasional hunger pang. It was waiting for the weight to come off once I realized that what I was doing was actually working. I have clear memory of complaining to one of my coworkers at the six-month and 60-pound mark that "I might go crazy before I take off the rest."

No matter how desperate I felt, I was careful not to let my impatience propel me toward taking more drastic measures (such as eating even less or taking diet pills). Diets that help you lose the weight unnaturally fast also help you gain it back just as fast. The problem with extremist dieting is that you're subscribing to a temporary behavior. I concentrated on the fact that my goal wasn't just to lose the weight but to find a method of accountability that I could commit to long term.

Staying Motivated

The term *motivation* when used in reference to dieting, is a temporary concept. It's a hope that you will be able to hang in there long enough to see a project through to completion. However, this wasn't just a project. I was trying to change my life permanently. Therefore, I needed something bigger than motivation. I needed a new perspective.

Instead of viewing weight loss (and the eventual maintenance of that weight loss) as a temporary state of existence, I viewed it as a series of continuous transactions. When I put forth an effort, I got something in return. My return on investment was either weight loss or not gaining it back. Even on the days when I didn't give a damn about what I ate, there was still a transaction going on.

If I ate 3,000 calories a day for five days, then I would gain 5 pounds. Therefore, I would simply make a better transaction the following week. There is no end to these transactions. It will continue going on for the rest of my life.

So what got me to pay attention?

Aside from the fact that I wanted to be healthier, I also wanted a better quality of life. I'm not just referring to physically functioning with greater ease, but I no longer wanted to resign myself to the same station in life. The one where I wouldn't allow myself to be a part of or enjoy something because of the weight.

Additionally, losing the weight became a symbolic act of defiance against societal expectations. The media love to run stories that preach "once fat, always fat." I was tired of hearing about studies that show "if you were an overweight child, you will be an obese adult" or "even if you lose the weight, you'll gain it back within two years."

The day I decided that I wasn't going to let those "facts" apply to me was the day my life changed.

The Joy of Discovery

I don't exactly recall when things such as fitting into my car or walking around the mall got easier. In fact, it was a lot like having a case of the hiccups, one second they were there and the next second, "Hey, they're gone!" However, when I finally recognized a breakthrough, I took time to appreciate it and give myself some credit. This was something I hadn't done the first time I lost weight. I was so obsessed with the end game of being skinny that I had never fully realized how far I had already come. This time I looked beyond just the weight loss and saw every breakthrough as a reason to celebrate.

Getting Closer

As I got closer to my goal weight, the small affirmation I made to myself about "never going back" became a concrete truth. Although, I discovered that it had less to do with not being heavy again and more to do with not going back to my old way of thinking. It was easy to keep my old destructive habits alive when losing weight meant I had to give up everything I loved and lead a life of drudgery.

Now, I knew I could eat the foods I desired and still be at the weight I desired. Now, I knew bad days could be corrected and momentary lapses in judgment weren't permanent failures unless I allowed them to be.

8

Just the Food Facts

Okay, folks, this is supposed to be where I shock and amaze you with my fabulous food choices. Actually, if that's what you are expecting, then you might want to stop reading now. As I mentioned earlier, I eat what I eat because it works for me and I'm happy with my decisions. I fully anticipate that some people will become critical while perusing my food choices and feel the need to point out that it lacks nutrients and is full of fat, sodium, and sugar.

If that's the case, then you may wonder why I'm willing to dangle myself in front of the firing squad. Truthfully, it's because I know many people are exactly like I was years ago. They feel as though they are stuck in a deep hole and the only way out means giving up the food they love. If something I share here can reach those people, then it was worth baring my food secrets. Also, I'm sharing this information with you because it's simply the truth. It's honestly what I eat on a regular basis.

A couple of relevant things I should mention before I go any further: I was 26 years old when I embarked on this journey. As I write this, I'm 31. I recognize that as the years move on, my body may change and I may not be able to eat these foods forever. Currently, I do not have high blood pressure or high blood sugar. Please remember, this is not me telling you to eat these meals, I'm simply sharing with you what I eat in a typical week.

Also, you will notice that I don't mention any beverages. Why? Because I only drink zero calorie beverages (such as diet soda, iced tea or water). I'm not a fan of coffee, alcohol or regular soda. You won't find any 400-calorie white chocolate espressos or 150-calorie cans of soda in my diet. In my humble opinion, why drink calories when you can eat them?

Here are meal examples for a typical week during my weight loss phase:

Monday:
- **Breakfast:** Kellogg's Special K Pastry Crisp – 100 calories
- **Lunch:** McDonald's McDouble (390) and Vanilla Ice Cream Cone (170) – 560 calories
- **Dinner:** 3 Hard Shell Tacos from Chipotle with chicken, cheese and sour cream – 605 calories
- **Daily Total:** 1,265 calories

Tuesday:
- **Breakfast:** Medium Banana – 105 calories
- **Lunch:** Del Taco Del Beef Burrito (490) and a Chocolate Chip Cookie (200) – 690 calories
- **Dinner:** McDonald's 10-Piece Chicken McNugget (470) and Vanilla Ice Cream Cone (170) – 640 calories
- **Daily Total:** 1,435 calories

Wednesday:
- **Breakfast:** Quaker Chewy Dipps Granola Bar – 140 calories

- **Lunch:** Subway Ham & Cheese 6-inch sub with light mayo (380) and a Double Chocolate Cookie (210) – 590 calories
- **Dinner:** 2 Wienerschnitzel Corn Dogs (250) – 500 calories
- **Daily Total:** 1,230 calories

Thursday:

- **Breakfast:** Kellogg's Special K Pastry Crisp – 100 calories
- **Lunch**: Burger King Double Cheeseburger (370) and a Chocolate Fudge Sundae (280) – 650 calories
- **Dinner:** KFC's Grilled Chicken Leg and Thigh, Mashed Potatoes, Gravy and Biscuit– 560 calories
- **Daily Total:** 1,310 calories

Friday:

- **Breakfast:** Quaker Instant Oatmeal Maple & Brown Sugar 1 Packet – 160 calories
- **Lunch:** El Pollo Loco's Beans, Rice and Cheese Burrito (430) and Chicken Leg (80) – 510 calories
- **Dinner:** Wendy's Jr. Bacon Cheeseburger (390) and 4-Piece Chicken Nuggets (180) – 570 calories
- **Daily Total:** 1,240 calories

Saturday:

- **Brunch:** IHOP "Two X Two X Two" (pancakes, eggs, sausage) with butter and sugar-free syrup – 680 calories
- **Dinner:** 2 Slices of DiGiorno Rising Crust "Three Meat" pizza (700) and Dreyer's Slow Churned Chocolate Light Ice Cream ½ cup (100) – 800 calories
- **Daily Total:** 1,480 calories

Sunday:

- **Breakfast:** Toast with butter – 200 calories

- **Lunch:** Subway Ham & Cheese 6-inch sub with light mayo (380) and a Double Chocolate Cookie (210) – 590 calories
- **Dinner:** McDonald's Quarter Pounder with Cheese (510) and Hot Fudge Sundae (330) – 840 calories
- **Daily Total:** 1,630 calories

Weekly Total: 9,590 calories (Daily average: 1,370)

Weight Loss vs. Maintenance Phase

As you can see from the examples, during my weight loss phase I was eating roughly 1,250 calories on the weekdays and then allowing myself a little more freedom over the weekends. When I'm in maintenance phase, I increase my daily caloric intake to about 1,800 calories a day, which is my current BMR. To this day, I still weigh myself at least once a week to see if I'm getting a little out of hand. If I gain 5 to 10 pounds, I immediately go back to 1,250 calories a day until I return to 170 pounds.

(A note regarding my goal weight: Although most height/weight charts state a woman of 5 feet 7 inches should weigh between 130 to 150 pounds, I didn't feel like turning into Rocky Balboa to power through losing another 20 pounds. My weight loss slowed down at the 170 pound mark, and I was happy there. The rest of the world may not be satisfied with that answer, but they don't live in my body, I do.)

Method to My Madness

Personal preference isn't the only reason most of my meals come from a drive-thru window. It also has to do with portion control, convenience and money. As I mentioned earlier, I like the fact that I can order something small that stays within my caloric budget and drive away.

Creating a path to success sometimes means identifying weaknesses and omitting them. For me, spending time around food and creating a large pot of something is an equation for eating more. It's like asking an alcoholic to your bartender for the evening. It's cruel and unusual punishment.

The less time I have to spend around food physically, the better. I don't feel there is any shame in trying to avoid your weaknesses. Our world is filled with temptations, so I strategize. If I can make mealtime a little easier on myself, then I do.

On the subject of convenience, I work full-time and I commute about three hours a day. I often eat dinner on the road; otherwise, I wouldn't be eating until after eight in the evening. Yes, I could find the time to prepare my meals over the weekend for easy reheating later, but as I've said before, that's just not me. I would rather spend the few hours it would take to plan, cook and portion my meals during the weekend by reading a book or watching a movie. It's important at the beginning of your journey to really evaluate your lifestyle and preferences and figure out what is going to make the most sense for you.

I'm a big fan of fast food restaurants' "dollar menus." These consist of smaller items, which also happen to be cheaper. I often spend less money on my lunch than my friends do on a coffee from Starbucks.

Food Proofing Your Home

Obviously, I don't live in a fast food bubble. I'm not always on the road and don't want to eat every meal out of my car. At some point, I have to go home and face my own kitchen. I also have to face the grocery store once a week and shop for other people. As much as I wish the rest of my loved ones were on board with my way of eating, that's just not reality.

You can't always control what other adults bring into the house or what you might have to feed your children. So, make sure that *you* are satisfied first. Keep portion-controlled amounts of the things you like to eat within reach. When it comes to snacking and side dishes, I have a "150 rule." If it is a non-trigger food that is available in 150-calorie portion sizes or less, it is probably already in my kitchen. For me, this includes granola bars, crackers, lunch-sized bags of chips, bananas, and a myriad of other "100 calorie" snack items.

So what do you do when you have to share mealtime with people not eating the same as you?

If you are the chef, pull a fast one. I will often substitute the regular ingredients of a meal with their lower-calorie counterparts and no one is the wiser. For instance, on taco night, I use leaner ground beef, low-fat refried beans and part-skim-milk cheese.

If you are not the chef and you're facing a gluttonous feast, keep the portion size of the highest calorie food on the small side and add something else on your plate to fill the void. Sometimes, mealtime is about picking the lesser of two evils. Eat an extra dinner roll if it helps you to leave the second helping of lasagna alone.

If all else fails, fly solo. I know it's not easy, but sometimes it's better to sit there with an entirely different plate of food so that you can stay on track. If everyone else is indulging in delivery pizza, go make yourself a sandwich. It's not that you can't eat the pizza, but chances are for the same amount of calories as two slices of pizza, you can have one hell of a sandwich with chips and a dessert.

When I do eat a solo meal at home, here are some of my staples:

- Grilled Cheese Sandwich with Kraft Cheese Single (260) and Progresso Clam Chowder (360) - 620 calories
- Tyson Chicken Patty (200) in Hamburger Bun (110) and Cheetos Individual 1-ounce bag (140) – 450 calories

- JimmyDean Delights Croissant Turkey Sausage, Egg White and Cheese sandwich (280), Doritos Individual 1-ounce bag (140) and Dreyer's Slow Churned Chocolate Light Ice Cream ½ cup (100) – 520 calories
- 4 ounces of Chunk Light Tuna (90) with 2 tbsp. Miracle Whip (80) on white bread (200) and Doritos Individual 1-ounce bag (140) – 510 calories

Weight Loss Markers

Throughout my 17-month journey down to 170 pounds, I documented the markers. Unlike other people, I had no rhyme or reason to how often I weighed myself. I just played it by ear. I would back off if I felt I was becoming too obsessed with the numbers. It took me a little over 10 months to lose 100 pounds, which means I was averaging about 10 pounds a month. The last 30 pounds took me another six months to lose. As expected, my weight loss began to taper off toward the end.

7/3/08 – 300 lbs.

8/3/08 – 283.6 lbs.

8/11/08 – 282.6 lbs.

8/15/08 – 280.8 lbs.

8/22/08 – 276.6 lbs.

8/29/08 – 274.4 lbs.

8/30/08 - 273.6 lbs.

9/5/08 – 272.8 lbs.

9/6/08 – 271.6 lbs.

9/20/08 – 269.2 lbs.

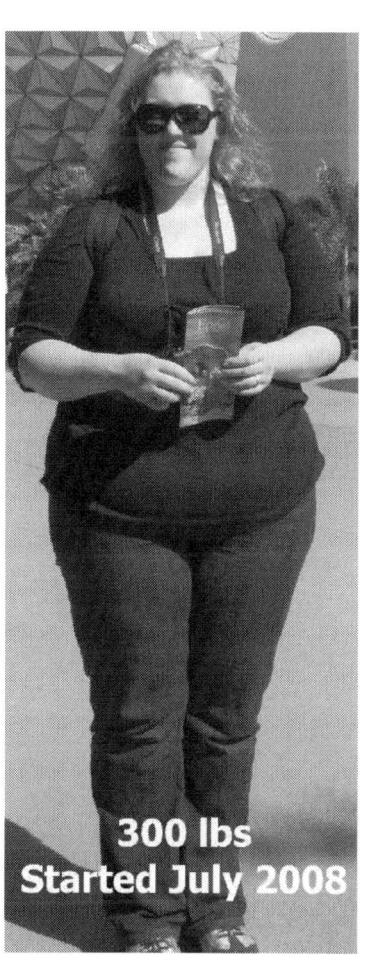

9/22/08 – 267.8 lbs.

9/26/08 – 267.2 lbs.

9/27/08 – 266.6 lbs.

10/8/08 – 264.2 lbs.

10/12/08 – 263 lbs.

➡

11/12/08 – 255 lbs.

11/13/08 – 254 lbs.

11/14/08 – 252.8 lbs

11/20/08 – 252 lbs.

11/21/08 – 250.8 lbs.

11/24/08 – 250 lbs.

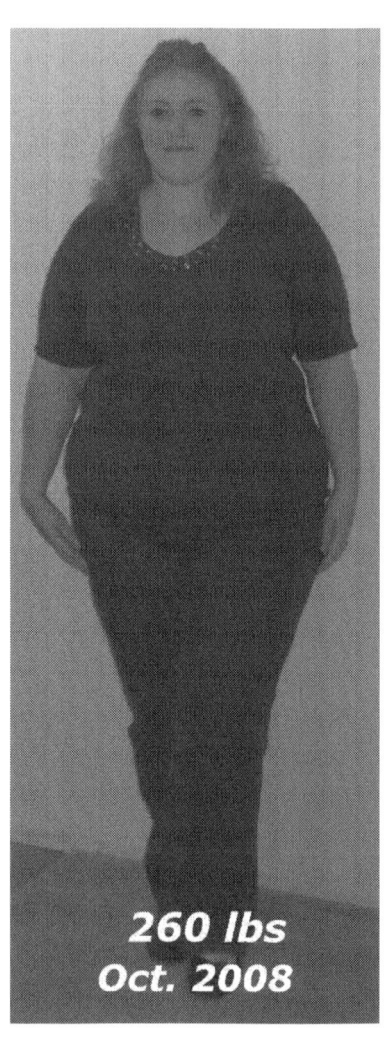

260 lbs Oct. 2008

11/26/08 – 249.4 lbs.

11/27/08 – 248.4 lbs.

12/1/08 – 248 lbs.

12/2/08 – 247.6 lbs.

12/3/08 – 246.6 lbs.

→ 12/7/08 – 245 lbs.

12/8/08 – 242.8 lbs.

12/17/08 – 239.8 lbs.

12/23/08 – 237.8 lbs.

12/24/08 – 236.6 lbs.

12/25/08 – 235.6 lbs.

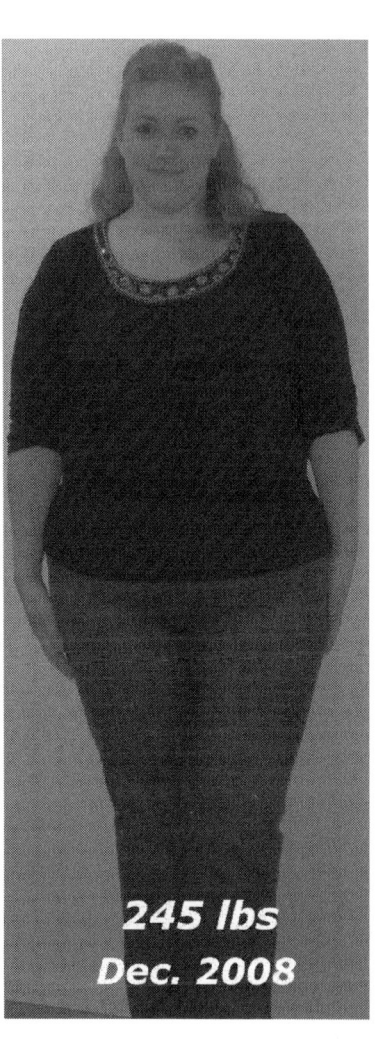

1/20/09 – 227.5 lbs.

1/28/09 – 226.6 lbs.

2/1/09 – 224.6 lbs.

2/4/09 – 222.4 lbs.

2/15/09 – 221.3 lbs.

2/16/09 – 219.8 lbs.

2/18/09 – 219.4 lbs.

2/22/09 – 217.6 lbs.

2/28/09 – 213.5 lbs.

3/15/09 – 208 lbs.

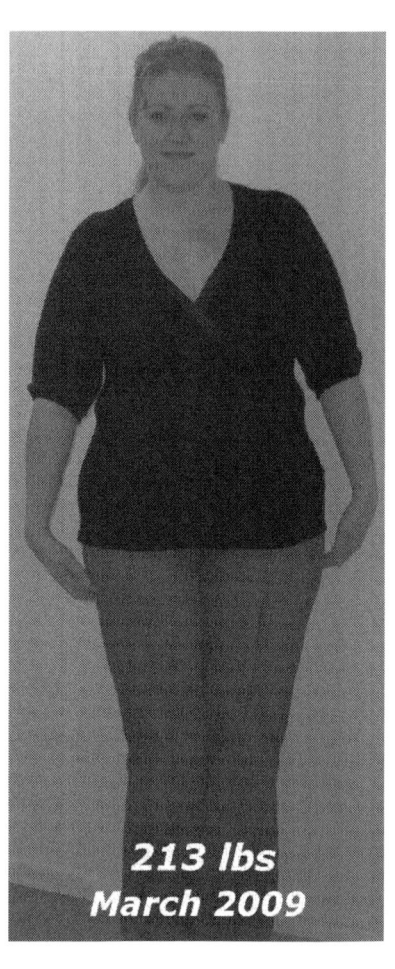

213 lbs March 2009

4/16/09 – 205 lbs.

5/14/09 – 199 lbs.

5/23/09 – 197.8 lbs.

5/29/09 – 194.4 lbs.

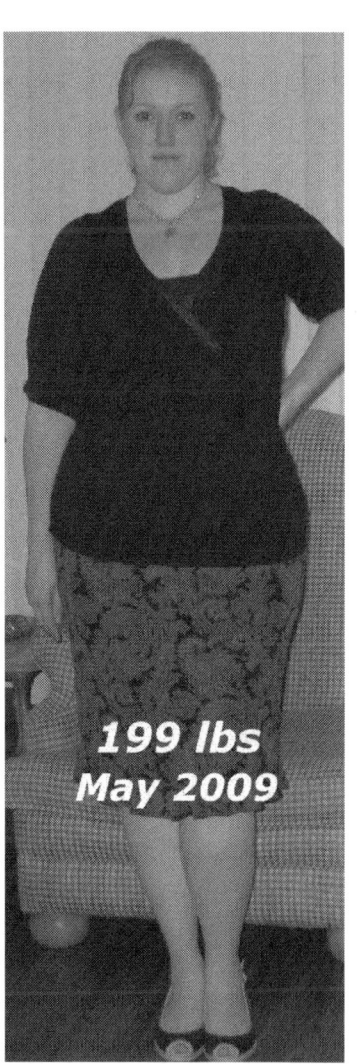

199 lbs May 2009

6/12/09 – 193.6 lbs.

7/25/09 – 185.2 lbs.

8/17/09 – 180.1 lbs.

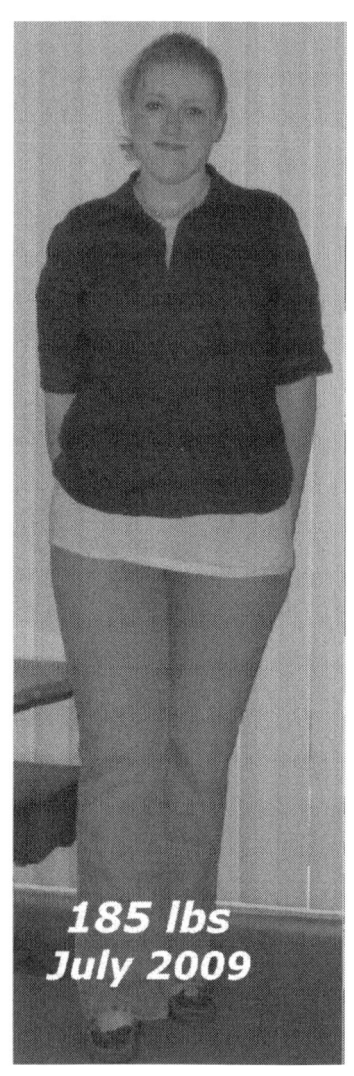

9/22/09 – 176.4 lbs.

10/14/09 – 173.8 lbs.

11/5/09 – 170 lbs.

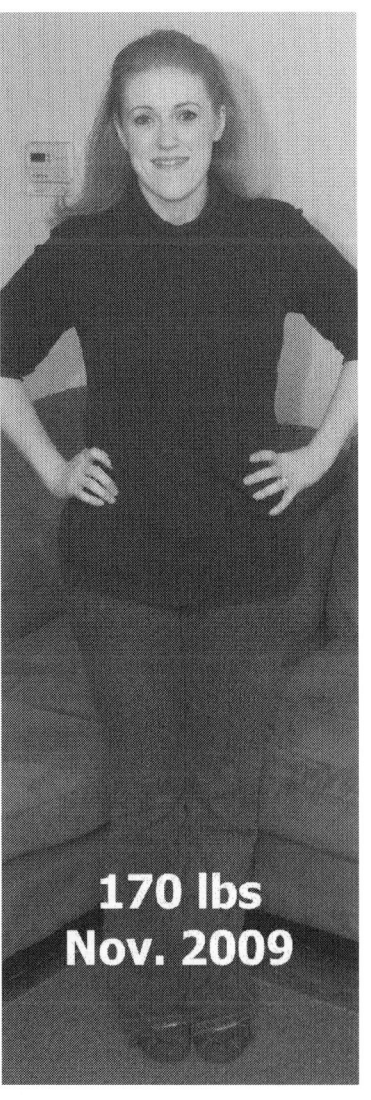

The Emotional Transformation: Confessions of a Food Addict

"I'm a food addict."
"I eat my emotions."

I had heard these statements many times from other people who struggled with the war on weight, but I never thought they applied to me. It's amazing how you don't think you have an emotional connection to food until one day you take away the very thing that's been numbing you for so many years.

On my long commute home from work each day, I would exit the I-210 and pull into a fast food joint (never the same one, of course, lest the person at the window recognize me) and order a large chocolate milkshake. This was not my breakfast, lunch or dinner. This was a "snack."

I was sucking an extra 800 to 1,200 calories a day through a straw! Then I would get home and eat dinner with my husband, which would be followed up by some over-the-top dessert. I was probably consuming 4,000 to 6,000 calories a day, easily. Remember, my BMR at this point was 2,500. So, hello, weight gain! However, those are just the numbers. The emotional repercussions of taking away my coping mechanism shook my world to its core.

Everyone is prepared to feel excited and wonderful when they first start losing weight, which you do, but for me, it was almost a superficial elation. It didn't remedy the fact that when I was stressed out and stuck in traffic for an hour and a half, every fiber of my being wanted to pull off the freeway and go grab a milkshake. This wasn't something that six cute little chicken nuggets was going to satisfy. My entire body was crying out for a half-dozen Krispy Kremes or something equally destructive.

It was in these moments that the real work began—in the quiet moments when I was alone, feeling negative emotions and had an overwhelming desire to gorge. This is what separates a true food addict from someone who just indulges occasionally. In those moments, my focus narrowed and I became fixated solely on my desire to eat. Through the fog and haze, I fought to remember the bigger picture. To remember why I was doing this, what I was trying to accomplish and what I was resigning myself to if I failed.

It's important to note here that sometimes you need help while trying to conquer the emotional side of this war (perhaps a dieting partner, support group or professional therapy). There is no shame in needing help. This is your journey and you need to create an environment for success.

The first few months of my new life were the most difficult and yet the most gratifying. I was fighting to form new eating habits and be accountable, but, at the same time, I was losing weight more rapidly than at any other time during my journey. It was a tenuous relationship. Fortunately, the freedom I was beginning to experience overshadowed the moments I was hungry (both literally and artificially).

I'm not exactly sure when it happened, but somewhere in the first few months, counting calories and eating smaller portions got easier. As I put more successful days behind me, my inner strength grew. The commitment to my new life, which was originally predicated on a stubbornness not to return to old ways, became an excitement for my future. By the time I had lost 50 pounds, people were starting to make comments about how different I looked, and their curiosity posed a hypothetical fork in the road for me.

Old Christine—the self-berating one—dictated that I downplay what I was doing and shy away from the attention. However, old Christine was the reason I had gained the weight in the first place, so I wasn't exactly inclined to listen to her anymore. I ended up doing the exact opposite of what old Christine would do, and I began posting my weight loss progress on the different social networking sites frequented by my friends and family. Ironically, putting myself out there became another tool for accountability.

The months to follow became a steady stream of choices that changed not only the way I had been eating, but also living. When I was spending time with friends and family, I made a conscience effort to stay out of my own head and be present in the moment. No more scanning the room to see if I was the largest person there. No more feeling bad about how I looked. I was there to spend time with people I cared about and that took center stage, not my self-doubt.

I started getting back to things I had remembered once enjoying, such as writing. Old Christine tried to do the "You're not good enough" song and dance, but she was no longer in charge. I prepared myself to "fake it 'til I make it" and made myself go through the motions of writing my first romance novel.

I began to take little leaps of faith, doing things I would never normally do: I shared samples of my writing with my coworkers even though I feared their rejection (something old Christine never would have done). I went bowling with my husband and friends despite my worry that everyone was looking at my big butt. I went to a salon and asked them to cut off my hair despite the self-doubt that told me I needed big hair to counter-balance my huge hips. I wore skirts and dresses on occasion even though the words *tree trunks* were dancing around in my head.

Looking back, I realize that my emotional transition to who I am right now took as much thought, determination, effort and faith as losing the weight did. For me, the two went hand in hand. I truly don't believe that one would have been possible without the other. The hardest part was not losing the weight but losing all the fear and self-hatred that had kept me from living my life.

10

The Whole Big (But Getting Smaller) Picture

I meet people every day who weigh 130 pounds. So it can be hard to wrap my brain around the fact that the amount of weight I lost actually equates to an average-sized woman or a small-framed man. In fact, it's something I try *not* to think about because it lures me into a mental jousting session over why I wasted so many years carrying around that extra "person."

My eagerness to put it all behind me is why I never started a blog, why I never kept a single pair of fat pants, why I don't like looking at old photos and why it took me years to write this book.

As much as I would like to, I can't run from my past. Reminders are everywhere. For those of us who have lost nearly half our body weight, one of the greatest reminders comes in the form of loose skin. Sadly, the only way to remove this skin is through body contouring and body lifting. These procedures can last seven to 10 hours, cost thousands of dollars and leave you with incisions spanning the length of whatever area you have worked on (torso, chest, upper arms or thighs).

Because I really don't want to be cut from stem to stern, I've had to learn to make peace with my body. I've had to make a conscious effort to concentrate on the positives and not the negatives.

Losing weight can be an absolute high, but like any new relationship, eventually the magic wears off. It may take a few years, but what was once a novelty can dissolve into "the norm."

Why am I telling you about this? Why am I not just concentrating on how great it is to lose 130 pounds? Because that's not the whole story. Because if I didn't tell you about some of the less attractive realities, you would only be getting half the picture and, frankly, not being honest about the whole picture is what makes the weight loss industry such a crock. The truth is, when the weight loss euphoria fizzles out, if you're not prepared to deal with the leftover emotions, it can destroy all you've worked so hard to accomplish.

Ups and Downs

It took a couple of years, but eventually my new body started to feel like the body I'd always had and old habits started to set in. The self-critiquing came back with a vengeance, along with my desire to numb out with food.

When people say weight loss maintenance is more difficult than losing it, this is what they are talking about: It's when you're past the point of being incentivized to stay on track by extreme weight loss or by the novelty of your new body and you're just left with, well ... you. This is why having a clear sense of who you are and what's important in life is a vital part of weight loss maintenance.

Those truths can act as an anchor when you're floating in a self-destructive fog. It wasn't until a couple of years after the weight loss that I came to the true realization that this whole changing my life thing was a marathon, not a sprint.

So have I magically weighed 170 pounds steadily since reaching my goal in November 2009?

No.

Does that make me a failure?

No.

The second "no" is actually more important than the first. Realizing I'm not a failure because I go up and down 5, 10 and even 15 pounds at times is important to making sure I don't gain it all back.

I realize for a person at an average healthy weight, the loss and gain of a few pounds is normal. For someone who has lost 100-plus pounds, it can feel like the end of the world. The problem is berating yourself over the gaining of a few pounds is a slippery slope. It can keep you in a dark place emotionally that makes you want to eat, which just leads to more weight gain. More dark. More food.

Addressing the problem for me starts mentally. I have to rationalize with myself. I'm human and life is filled with stress, anxiety, holidays, family drama and other events and emotions that can cultivate the coping mechanism of overeating. I can't address the behavior of overeating until I've let the guilt associated with it go. So I write about it or I talk about it with people I trust. What I don't do is let it go unacknowledged. If I do, the guilt will turn into a cancer that spans beyond a day or a week and, before you know it, six months has gone by and the 100 pounds is back.

Once I've rationalized with myself that what I've done is *not* Armageddon and I've successfully purged some of the emotional guilt, I try to analyze the actual behavior. Have I been eating more after work? Have I been eating more after dealing with a certain family member or a friend? If I didn't gain the weight because of a temporary event, such as a vacation, then it's due to a deeper issue.

If I can find the stressor, then I can consciously decide to handle it another way. I pay special attention to whether or not I'm actually hungry. For me, feeling a strong emotion on an empty stomach can result in me inhaling a tray of brownies. Instead of reaching for what I'm craving, I force myself to eat an actual meal. After that, I turn to an activity that keeps me busy. Whether it's reading, writing, cleaning the house, going to the movies, or shopping.

Of course, trying to resolve the core issue is recommended, but depending on the situation, the stressor may be out of your control. Sometimes the only thing you have control over is how you react and deal with that stress.

Body Distortion

I used to pride myself on having a realistic body image. I thought when it came to clothing I knew what I could get away with and what I could not. I carefully chose items that covered me fully but didn't look like a potato sack.

Then I lost 100 pounds and everything changed.

I would catch a glimpse of my reflection in a window and I would have to do a double take. I couldn't believe it was me! Girl Scout's honor, this truly wasn't a case of me marveling at how "good" I looked. My brain was genuinely out of sync with my physical appearance.

As it turns out, this phenomenon (thinking you are larger than you actually are) is experienced by most who have lost a substantial amount of weight. I have yet to meet or read about someone who has lost 100 or more pounds who didn't experience body distortion on some level.

The true danger comes when you can't see the difference between the distortion and reality. When you look in the mirror and you still feel the very same way about yourself as you did before you lost the weight. This can be a real condition called Body Dysmorphic Disorder (BDD) and it is important to seek professional help.

For me, the intense shock I felt when I would accidentally see myself softened over time, but it never went away fully. I still have moments when I think I'm bigger than I actually am.

Recently, I spent the entire day in a dress. Something I never do. Since I only anticipated being in that dress for a few hours for a special event, I put a pair of jeans and a sweater in my car to change into afterward.

Then a friend asked me to hang out after the event. I tried to think of a way I could excuse myself, run to my car, grab the clothes and change in the bathroom without seeming like a freak, but alas, I wasn't that creative. So I stayed in the dress all day while we ran around the mall and had dinner at a nearby restaurant.

By the end of the night, old habits were flaring up, and I had a picture of jiggly thighs and huge hips dancing around in my head. I tried to ignore the invading insecurities and thought I was doing pretty well until I got home and saw myself in a full-length mirror. I immediately recognized that the girl in the mirror was not the huge image I had in my head.

To this day, I still struggle with the lingering effects of a distorted body image. The only difference now is that I know my thinking (not my body) is distorted.

The Lighter Side

Life can be funny at times and in the months and years following my weight loss I've found having a sense of humor is priceless.

People's Reactions

First, let me say that the majority of the reactions I have received since starting this journey have been overwhelmingly positive. I am truly humbled by the support and love from family and friends. However, I never expected some of the reactions I received to be quite as peculiar or as humorous as they were.

The Stalker: One day I found myself in a part of town where I used to work. I decided to pick up some stuff at a nearby grocery store. I was walking down the cereal aisle when I had this nagging feeling that someone was watching me. I quickly turned, only to find one of those displays in the middle of the aisle holding boxes of frosted cereal that was on sale. So I wrote it off as me being paranoid and kept shopping. The feeling returned when I was looking at TV dinners in the freezer section. I could swear I saw a man peeking around a corner at me through the freezer door I was holding open, but when I shut it, he was gone. Finally, in the soda aisle, a man cleared his throat from behind me and I turned around to find an old coworker. He was very nice, but admitted to following me around for the last 15 minutes trying to figure out if I was, "the girl [he] used to work with."

The "Bigger Girl": One of the most surreal experiences I have had since losing the weight was when I had to return to the place that capped off my original descent to rock bottom. The business trip I described earlier is actually an annual event. I returned to this event exactly one year later and 100 pounds lighter. Generally, the same people attend the event each year, and their reactions (if any) to me varied. Some didn't notice a difference, some people noticed right away, some looked uncomfortable but asked, "Is there something different about you?" and then some thought I was an entirely different person. Over the course of one week, I had at least a dozen people ask me, "What happened to the bigger girl that was here last year?" I just smiled and said, "Oh, you mean me?"

The "Are you ill?" Reaction: This one actually breaks my heart a little. It makes me wonder what kinds of things people have experienced in their own lifetime that they automatically assume when someone has experienced a dramatic weight loss, it's because they have become seriously ill. I was at another event for work when an older volunteer came up and hugged me for what seemed to be an awkward length of time. Throughout the event, the volunteer would look over at me and smile. I was beginning to worry something bad was happening. Did I have a giant pimple on my face? Was my boss going to lay me off? It wasn't until after the meeting that I found out from a coworker that this volunteer had thought I was sick. He had actually approached her and asked about my dire diagnosis.

It took her a minute to figure out what he was referring to, then laughed and told him I had simply lost weight.

Some Things Never Change

When you lose a substantial amount of weight, you expect your life will change. However, I was shocked to find that some things didn't change at all. My heavier alter ego spent so much time blaming personal fears and frustrations on being overweight that it was an epiphany to find some things stayed the same.

Clothes Shopping: I thought it was hard to shop for clothes simply because of my size. I used to hate shopping in "plus size clothing stores" where they charge you two to three times more per item and where shopping for a pair of jeans is like being stuck in an episode of *Sesame Street*. You have to find the color/shape/letter that directly corresponds to the curvature of your butt. Don't get me wrong, every woman (and man) should have a place where they can find flattering, fashionable clothes. I just never chalked my frustrations up to being a woman or the fashion industry. I now know that sizing makes no sense, anywhere! I'm a size 10 in one store and a size 14 in another. I can grab two pairs of pants from the same manufacturer, same size, and one will be too tight in the tummy with a "saggy butt" appearance in the back, while the other is too tight in the thighs and gives me a bad case of camel toe in the front (look it up if you don't know).

High Heels: Once a klutz, always a klutz. Couldn't walk in them before, still can't now.

Rock Climbing and Rollercoasters: I might have felt as if I was ready to take on the world following the weight loss, but not heights. I went indoor rock climbing with a friend after I lost the weight thinking how awesome it would be to experience an activity I wouldn't have been able to do before. Yeah, not so much. I got halfway up the wall and started shouting, "Get me down, get me down, get me down."

Spray Tanning: Call me narrow-minded, but I always thought of spray tans (or tanning, in general) as a skinny girl sport. It was something I would never do because I was normally hiding under enough layers of clothing to make an Eskimo sweat. All that changed when I was asked to be a bridesmaid. The dresses we were going to be wearing were strapless and ended right above the knee. Now, if you didn't notice in any of my pictures, I am Casper-white! As in, nearly transparent, blue-vein white. So for the first time in my life, I was in dire need of a tan.

I did my research and decided to go with the kind of spray tan where you stand inside a booth (a little larger than a shower) and a deceivingly pleasant female voice does a countdown. From there you are power-hosed (excuse me, airbrushed) with tanner in a side-to-side sweeping motion. They tell you it's okay to breathe in the mist, but you should try not to. Of course, I panicked as if someone was trying to waterboard me and literally gulped for air the second the spray was just below my mouth. I was so traumatized by the experience, I thought I was going to have a heart attack. Somehow, despite my panic, I still convinced myself to turn around and let the jets do my back so I wouldn't look like a two-toned Twinkie. I came out of the booth shaking like a poodle pulled from freezing flood waters. Needless to say, spray tanning wasn't my thing before and it's not my thing now.

Copyright Concerns

By far, the most bizarre thing that has happened to me since I started this journey was when I discovered that a Bulgarian company was selling their diet pills using *my* "before-and-after" photo. The picture was ripped off from my website (www.christineleo.com) and used without my permission.

In March 2013, I was contacted by a suspicious consumer of the diet pills who decided to run an image search on my photo and found my website with my real story. If it weren't for him, I would have never known. I've since run my own image search and have found that my picture is being used in reference to the same diet pill on multiple websites in different languages.

Sadly, after doing quite a bit of research, I've come to find I have no recourse. If it was an American-based company, I could send them a request for photo credit, a take-down notice, a cease-and-desist letter or hire a lawyer and file suit. All of which, most likely, would produce no results, except for the last method, which could be costly. Most articles state that if the infringer is in a foreign country, it's not worth my time or energy.

Below is the before-and-after photo that used without my consent.

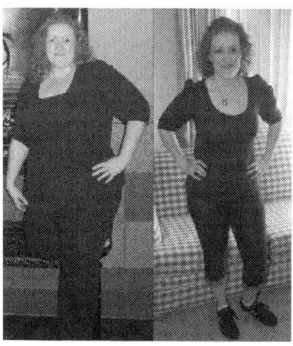

On the left: Me in July 2008 at 300 pounds.

On the right: Me in 2011 at 170 pounds.

Yes, There's Life after Losing

Today, life is better, but not perfect.
Like many who have walked this road, I put weight loss on a pedestal. I was convinced that if only I could lose weight, everything in my life—internally and externally—would come together. I thought my self-confidence would do a complete 180. I would be so naturally positive that the other parts of my life would fall into place because I had finally conquered my one, true demon.

I was wrong.

Losing the weight didn't mean I lost the deeply ingrained "glass-half-empty" perspective that I had been battling my whole life. It just meant I lost my scapegoat. I could no longer blame my unhappiness on the weight. I had to confront my genuine self and find a new definition of happiness.

The Real Deal

So now that you know your fairy godmother won't be fluttering down from the clouds with a magic wand and making all your troubles poof into oblivion, let's talk about what you can expect should you undertake a journey like mine:

- **Increased freedom:** The anchor of the physical weight will be gone.
- **Increased self-belief:** You will learn what you are truly capable of achieving.
- **Increased clarity:** By losing weight, you will be clearing a path to the real you.
- **Increased quality of life:** Whether from a heightened sense of well-being or from the ability to function with greater ease, your quality of life will improve.

How do you know when you are ready?

At the risk of being annoyingly vague: You'll just know. The key for me was hitting rock bottom. You have to be *truly* fed up. If there is any part of you that honestly feels that the way you are currently living your life is acceptable, you will not commit to a new way of life for the long term. You might give it a try, but the second something makes you a little uncomfortable, you'll run back to what you used to know. You have to be at a point where there is no longer a choice about changing your life.

How do you start?

First, don't overthink it and stress yourself out. There's no special day or way to start. All that matters is that you actually start. It can be your next meal or the next day. Simply do something different. Remember that everything you are currently doing, with regard to eating and activity level, have led you to where you are now. They keep you in your current state of existence and are most likely propelling you toward something far worse with each passing day. All you need to do is shake things up by making one positive change.

If you are reading this now because you are currently at a station in life where you are fed up, there is hope. Time is an eternally moving train and every minute of every day is an opportunity for you to hop aboard and leave your current station behind. The price of admission is that you simply make a positive change. Ultimately, the days, weeks, months and years will go by, whether you remain where you are or hop aboard to see where the journey takes you.

Why I'm Grateful for My Journey

Physically: I can move in ways I couldn't before. I can keep up with the average person and not feel as if I'm cloaked in an anvil of weight that keeps me from functioning and breathing freely.

Mentally: I don't have the same fog of self-doubt constantly screwing with my perception of reality, and when it creeps back in, I can identify it as distorted.

Emotionally: I'm more balanced than I was before. I no longer feel that I'm on some dark and isolated island where nobody understands my pain. I took the ferry off that island a while ago and began to reacquaint myself with loved ones.

Spiritually: I recognize that there is a higher power, without which none of this would be possible. My inner strength, clarity and focus must have come from something benevolent because I was so low when I started this journey, I feel it's a miracle that I'm even here to type this sentence.

In conclusion, there is no conclusion. I will be doing this dance for the rest of my life. No matter the method for my weight loss madness, ignorance is no longer an option. If I gain the weight back, it will be because I choose to. I will be carrying this bag the rest of my life. But, hey, it's a heck of a lot lighter than the bag I used to carry.

About the Author

Christine Leo was born and raised in Southern California where she currently resides with her tech-savvy husband. When she's not eating fast food or stuck in traffic, you'll find her completely engrossed in a romance novel or writing one. Christine holds a BA in Communications, which would have been Creative Writing had the universe simply dropped a novel on her head a little sooner. A heavy one.
At least 600 pages. Hard cover.

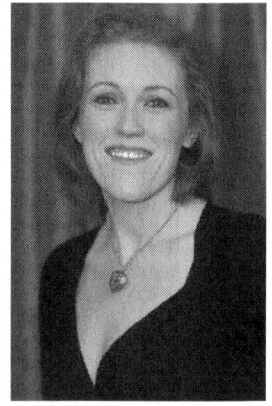

Visit Christine Leo online at:
www.ChristineLeo.com
www.VeggiesNotIncluded.com

Made in the USA
Lexington, KY
19 July 2014